My Past Is Now My Future

A Practical Guide to Dementia Possible Care©

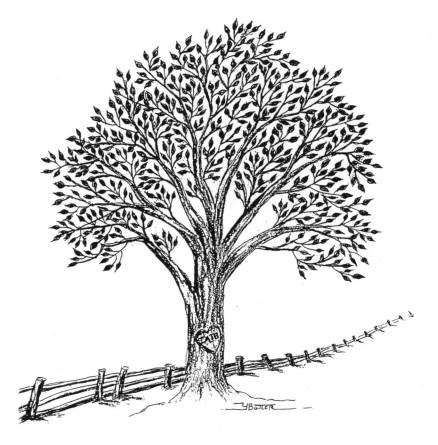

Lanny D. Butler, MS, OTR

Kari K. Brizendine, PT

My Past Is Now My Future

© 2005

Lanny D. Butler
Kari K. Brizendine

ISBN 1890306819
Library of Congress Control Number: 2005924197

Cover artwork and illustrations
by Yvonne E. Butler of Cavalier, North Dakota

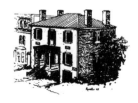

Warwick House Publishing
720 Court Street
Lynchburg, VA 24504

Dedication

This book is dedicated to all the individuals who have been diagnosed with dementia, who have shared their joys and sorrows, and allowed us to share a small part of their lives.

We dedicate this book to the families and care-givers who, through their actions on a daily basis, demonstrate the love and support they feel for each individual under their care.

Finally, this book is dedicated to our families who provided love and support to us as we attempted to put into words the joy we continue to feel each day as we interact with people with dementia.

Lanny D. Butler

Kari K. Burgendin

Contents

Living with Dementia
How perception becomes reality
(from Lanny's perspective)

What we perceive to be true becomes our reality. If we believe that an individual who has dementia is unable to bathe, dress, feed, and toilet themselves, that will become your loved one's reality, only because you have made it so for them. Often, we unknowingly take away these abilities, out of love, but also out of ignorance of what can be done. By doing for them, we have taken away their ability to participate in life and have taken away much joy we could have shared together.

This book is our attempt to provide you an alternative to caring for your loved one. Using the stages of dementia developed by B. Reisburg in his Global Deterioration Scale, we will attempt to change your perception of the process of dementia and thereby change your reality of what is possible in the months and years ahead. We call our approach to living with dementia, Dementia Possible Care©.

The Day I Won the Lottery
Entering the reality of the demented individual
(from Kari's perspective)

Many frustrating days were spent trying to get my clients with dementia to follow my directions. "Nora, place the walker in front of you and take two steps" or "Jim, sit down and rest five minutes." It just wasn't working. Nora would be rearranging the furniture or Jim would be pacing up and down the hall. No amount of repeated direction or gesture worked. I even tried to sound firm in my command. "Sadie, stand up from the chair." Sadie would unlock her brakes and roll down the hall. My first thought would be I can't do anything with these people. They have dementia. I need to be working with people I can change, people who will listen to me and do what I say.

Then one day the heavens opened and all that was not possible became possible. I learned from my mentor, Lanny Butler, that I had it all wrong. Rather than expecting people to enter my reality, suppose I would decide to enter theirs! What do you mean by entering their reality? The things they are doing just don't make sense to me. Why would Elsie be layering up her clothes? One sweater is enough. Why would Walter walk down the hall polishing the woodwork? It's already shiny and clean. Furthermore, why would Oscar have a bowel movement in the trashcan when the toilet is right behind that door? Enter their reality? Are you nuts?

"Kari, first of all, Elsie has a disease process that has destroyed her hypothalamus, an area of the brain programmed for temperature regulation. She perceives that she is freezing cold most of the time. Walter used to be a janitor at the elementary school and he kept everything in immaculate condition in spite of the kids destroying it moment by moment. As for Oscar, he has no clue that the toilet is behind that door, which is identical to the adjacent closet door, so he has found the next best place."

The light bulb went on in my head and thoughts of my past, present, and future attempts with the dementia population flashed before me.

"And Annie—she's not trying to escape from the unit when she stands in the doorway?"

"Correct, she has forgotten how to turn around."

"And Frank is not taking his shoes off for attention?"

"No, he's feeling pain because of the bunions on his feet."

"And Myrtle is not hoarding everyone else's clothes?"

"No, she used to work in a clothing store and it was her responsibility to hang up the clothing. "

"And Nettie walking down the hall with Sadie's underwear on her head... is just wearing the night cap that she has worn to bed for the past sixty years!"

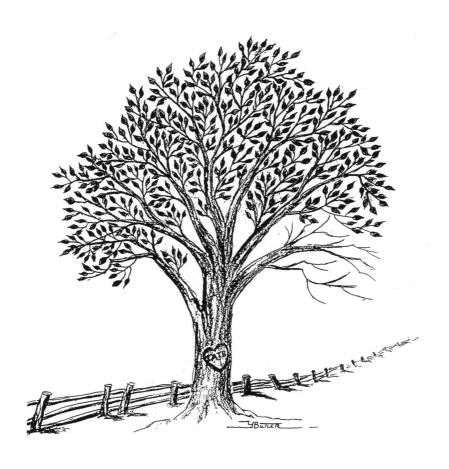

STAGE 1

It seems that whenever I have an important meeting I just can't leave the house on time. It started just like any other morning. The alarm was set to ring thirty minutes early. I got out of bed and into the shower only to realize that I had forgotten to get a washcloth. Dripping water through the bedroom to the hall closet, I grabbed a washcloth and went back to the shower. I toweled off and tried three pair of pantyhose before I found the ones with no runs in them. I dressed the kids, fed them, packed lunches, gathered homework and sent them off to school. It's twenty minutes to meeting time with a fifteen-minute commute and I can't find the damn car keys. I searched the entire house, papers flew, pillows were shoved, door locks were checked, coat pockets were turned inside out.

Stage 1

Did you know that short-term memory loss is one of the primary symptoms of stress? And it seems that the more stress there is in your life the worse your memory becomes.

About fifteen years ago, due to a reorganization of the state hospital system, the hospital where I was working was scheduled to close. After almost twelve years of living in the same community, my wife, children, and I decided to move 1300 miles away from friends and family and start a new life in Charlottesville, Virginia.

It has been said that moving is one of the greatest stressors in life. Everything changes. New job, new address, new phone number, finding your way around a new city, and learning where to find everything. One of the most difficult changes for me was finding a new doctor. Now, I consider myself a very down to earth, practical person, so my approach to locating a new physician went something like this. I asked everyone I worked with whom they saw, and found two co-workers who said I should try Dr. Dan Sawyer, as he was very thorough and took our insurance. (Both great reasons it seemed to me at the time.) As I had not had a physical in about ten years, and I needed one for my new job, I made an appointment with Dr. Sawyer. Little did I know that this decision would change the direction of my professional life.

Dr. Dan, as I now call him, went through all the normal routine parts of a physical exam: EKG, temperature, BP, height, weight, pulse, urinalysis, and routine blood work, but he then said something that no other doctor had ever mentioned before. He said, "I need to get a BASELINE on your memory. I want you to remember these three words and the following number." As he was making this request he walked over to the drawer next to the sink and began to put on a pair of rubber gloves. For a male, the most stressful part of a physical is when the doctor checks your prostate. And, of course, Dr. Sawyer chose at that moment to provide me with the three words and the following number: 8235101. Something I have never been able to do is remember numbers. Have you ever noticed that at the mall there is never a phone book next to a working telephone, and across the mall at the phone that is out of order is a brand new phone book chained in place? I am the guy that will look up the number and continue to repeat it as I cross the mall until I get about ten feet from the working phone and realize that I have forgotten the number. Well, on the third attempt, I write the number on my hand so that I will have it when I get to the working phone. Most people who know me realize that I have problems remembering numbers as every day my hands are covered in ink by midmorning. So when Dr. Dan asked me what was the number backwards ten minutes after checking my prostate, my reply was, "What number? I can't remember it forwards." He than repeated the number for me and my strategy was to repeat the number forward and enunciate the last digit, and repeat the number and enunciate the second to last digit and so on until the entire number was recreated backwards. He then asked me what were the three objects he had asked me to remember, and I was able to get two out of the three. Dr. Dan then made a statement that changed my life. He said, 'Stress can cause you to have problems with new learning and remembering this new information after only a short period of time. In order for me to know if you are having problems with your memory I must obtain a baseline of how you deal with new learning, what strategies you use, and how well you retrieve new information under stress. Now I know your strategies, so next year when you have your physical I will be able to determine if your short-term memory has changed, if your strategies continue to work for you, or if further testing is necessary to determine if what we are seeing is early dementia.'

During the first stage of the Global Deterioration Scale you see no symptoms other than the memory problems we all have when we are under stress.

"My Way"

Each of us is unique with our own individual way of doing things. Most of us go about our lives completing complex tasks without thinking about how we are doing them; we do them at a subconscious level. An example of this behavior is driving a car. Initially, we are conscious of every movement of our hands on the steering wheel and every time we place our foot on the brake. We are acutely aware of the vehicle behind us and how far away from the back of our car they are driving. Eventually you stop thinking and acting in this manner, and driving becomes subconscious except when we are in unusual circumstances such as a new traffic pattern, or driving on an unfamiliar highway, congestion on the road, or the road conditions change.

Most of us are unaware that we complete our daily routines in much the same manner. Our routine is unique to us; no two individuals have the same routine, nor do they complete the same tasks in a like manner.

My morning routine is unique only to me. I tend to wake up between four and five o'clock every morning. I get out of bed, go to the bathroom, then stumble into the kitchen and make a pot of coffee. After drinking about ten cups of coffee, I return to the bathroom and shave and shower. Notice I said shower; I do not take baths if I can help it. I choose not to use a washcloth; I have always considered them to be a total waste of material. Rather, I shower with a bar of soap. Holding the bar of soap in my right hand, I lather my left shoulder and then proceed to the rest of my body. The order of body parts bathed is unique to me; I do not think about what I will wash next; rather, the entire process is subconscious to me.

Why is this important? As an occupational therapist, it is my responsibility to enable my patients to be as independent as possible in completing their self-care. This usually occurs with use of adaptive methods or equipment. Generally, I request my clients to start at the head and progress towards their feet. If my client has a dementing disease, and this is not the unique order or way this individual has always completed his bath or the sequence of how he dresses, it is new learning…something that he is unable to complete or has extreme difficulty with. The individual will follow my verbal cues and wash the body parts on command but will tend not to sequence through the task, resulting in a very long process. Often this person will be bathed or dressed by others, as the caregiver believes the individual no longer has the ability to do so for himself.

We now realize that by knowing the individual's "way" of completing these tasks, the basic set-up and where they start the process, is enough to allow them to independently sequence through the task. We also know that those activities learned early in life tend to be the last activities people with dementia will lose. Therefore, it is possible for people with dementia to continue to bathe and dress, and remain continent well into the last stages of dementia.

Most of "My Way" of doing things is known only to me. Even though I have been married over twenty-eight years, my wife knows little of my morning routine. Why? Because most of these activities are done in isolation. Do you know how many squares of toilet paper your spouse or loved one uses? Do they fold it before they use it; do they stand up before wiping? Although this may seem irrelevant, each individual routine becomes subconscious and tends to occur exactly the same way every day and every time.

Although it in no way answers all the questions, we have included a survey to assist you in gathering this important information. (See Appendix 1) We have named this questionnaire "My Way." We strongly suggest you fill out the questionnaire and place it somewhere safe, as it will be worth its weight in gold to future caregivers and therapists when you no longer can explain your way of doing activities and your personal preferences.

Natural Aging vs. Dementia

Over twenty-five years ago I was sitting in class at the University of North Dakota and a very wise professor made a profound statement in her lecture. It went something like this. 'If you don't know what to expect in natural aging, how will you know if what you are seeing in your occupational therapy assessments is unusual or significant?' Fifteen years later as I was preparing a lecture on aging, I was going through a box of my old books and papers and found my notes of that lecture and realized for the first time how profound this statement had been. Her choice of words was excellent, she did not use the term Normal Aging; rather she used the term Natural.

Natural aging is what occurs to everyone irrespective of cultural differences, gender, or chronic disease. There are several generalized changes associated with natural aging that by their very nature have all-encompassing effects on the individual's overall function. The first change is a loss of elasticity and pliability of tissues. The effects of these changes are found in all body systems, including the musculoskeletal, cardiovascular, and pulmonary.

As the individual ages, there is a change in the ratio of fat and water in the body. The decrease in body water results in increased viscosity of mucous secretions, decreased saliva production, decreased eye lubrication, decreased intestinal mobility, and decreased sweat production.

The third change that affects multiple symptoms is an increase in the time it takes to respond to a stimulus. For example, an increased time for your eyes to accommodate to changes in light conditions, a decrease in heart rate, and increase in the amount of time for food to go through the digestive tract.

Probably the one fact that everyone accepts about the brain and aging is that adults lose thousands of brain cells each day and brain cells do not regenerate at a speed capable of affecting dementia at this time. The brain reaches its maximum weight at age twenty and shows a progressive loss of weight throughout the natural aging process. Current research indicates that loss in brain weight in otherwise healthy older adults does not lead to a decrease in intellectual function. Impaired thought processes are not an expected change with age. It has been further noted in research that while performance on practical problem solving tasks appears to peak in the middle years, the level of performance of sixty and seventy-year olds is essentially the same as that of twenty-year olds.

What my wise professor stated over twenty-five years ago still holds true today. If you don't know what to expect in natural aging, how will you determine if what you are seeing is significant and unusual? It is our attempt to provide clues of what is happening throughout the dementing process and, with this identification, provide practical possibilities to assist you and your family in dealing with the physical and cognitive changes that will occur.

Dementing Diseases

One of the most often asked questions is what is the difference between Alzheimer's disease and dementia. Dementia is a global term for the loss of cognitive and memory function. To be diagnosed with dementia, at least two spheres of mental activity must be impacted showing deterioration. These spheres include memory, language, orientation, perception, attention, and the ability to carry out purposeful tasks. No single test can identify a specific dementia. Generally, ruling out all other curable and incurable causes of memory loss completes a diagnosis. There are about seventy forms of dementia. Alzheimer's disease is the most common form of irreversible dementia. It is estimated that approximately 50 percent of diagnosed cases of dementia will be classified as Alzheimer's disease. A true diagnosis of Alzheimer's disease can only be made after an autopsy of the brain, though current diagnoses are accurate over 90 percent of the time. During the autopsy the brain is noted to be smaller and a different shape than the average brain. There are tangles and plaques present in the brain and the areas of the brain that hold short-term memory, ability to understand incoming information, language ability, the ability to remember, and total personality are affected.

Multi-infarct dementia is the second largest group of dementing diseases. It is felt that approximately 5 percent of all cases fall into this classification. Multi-infarct dementia is very similar in pathology to CVA or stroke. It is often the result of a long history of coronary artery disease. In the past this disorder was often called "hardening of the arteries." The deficits are a result of a number of large and small lesions in the brain tissue. These areas may be spread over the surface of the brain, be more localized or closer together. Location of these lesions will dictate the symptoms. A step-by-step decline, fluctuating speed of progression, and periods of improvement mark the course of multi-infarct dementia. Personality is usually preserved. This type of dementia is more commonly diagnosed in men.

Reisburg, in his Global Deterioration Scale, has divided the progression of dementia into seven stages for assessment of primary degenerative dementia. It takes careful observation to determine the degree of decline or stage of dementia. The signs and symptoms will vary slightly from one individual to another. The speed of deterioration will vary by individual and type of disease, with some individuals plateauing at a given stage for months or even years. Others progress through the seven stages without a plateau occurring. It may help you to conceptualize these stages of decline by thinking about the growth and development of an individual. Dementia is this developmental process in reverse. The last things learned (higher cognitive skills, judgment, tact) are the first skills lost. By knowing what occurs at each level we can predict behavior and develop strategies to enable individuals to continue to function in their environments despite cognitive loss.

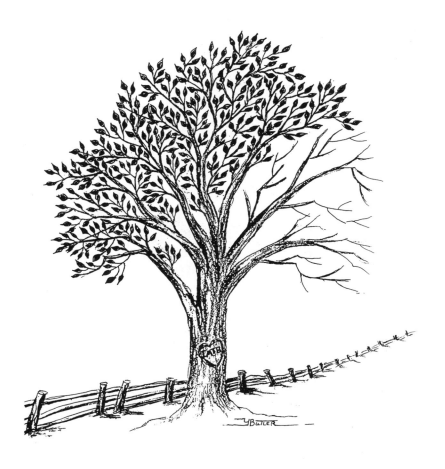

STAGE 2

I've bought cases of post-it notes.
"Turn off your headlights…"
"Lock the back door…"
"Check the stove…"

I keep them in my day planner. No one sees them but me. I send myself voicemails to remember names, projects, meetings, and I make lists. Sometimes I have lists for my lists. Extra time, extra planning, and reminders keep everything in order. Something is terribly wrong but no one knows but me.…

Stage 2

All of us have a problem remembering some things sometimes. How we deal with these short-term memory losses—our compensatory strategies—are unique and a part of us. However, these strategies will become our first line of defense throughout the first three stages of the Global Deterioration Scale if the cause of our memory problems is something other than stress.

My wife is a list maker; she makes lists about her lists. As she completes each task she will check it off her list (something she appears to gain great pleasure from). She makes lists for me, and again as I complete each task, she checks it off my list. I tend not to make lists; I usually fly by the seat of my pants. However, my compensatory strategy was to marry Diane. For over twenty-eight years she has kept me on track, making sure I remembered important appointments and commitments.

People who enter Stage 2 of the Global Deterioration Scale find short-term memory loss is occurring more frequently. Compensatory strategies are developed that work. An example of a compensatory strategy for individuals who must take medication several times a day might be setting up their medications in sectioned pill cases, which allows them to visually monitor if they have taken their necessary medication. Pill cases have been developed that are on a timer and ring or signal when it is time to take the next dose of medication. For those who can't remember if they have taken their medications and risk an overdose by retaking that medication, medication boxes have also been developed which unlock only at designated times.

Generally during this stage no one knows that the individual is having memory problems. Their spouse doesn't know, their children don't know, their co-workers have no idea because their compensatory strategies are working. People functioning in this stage will get up, go to work on time, do a good day's work, have a great social life (if they ever had one), drive. In other words, they continue to live their lives independently. They are functioning independently because they have become so good at dealing with their short-term memory losses through external aids.

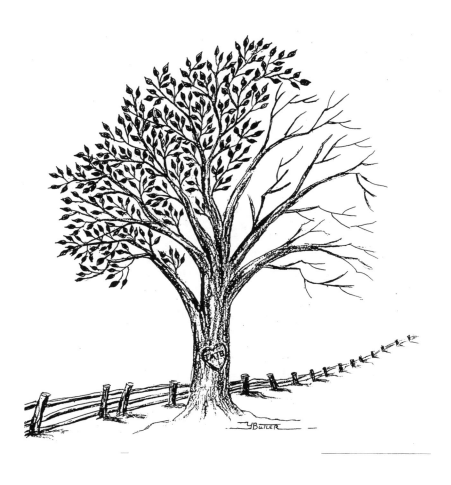

STAGE 3

I'm panicking; I know something is terribly wrong.

I don't know what to do but cover when I screw up.

I asked my secretary for an important file, then one hour later asked again. She had already given it to me.

I laughed and said I had really not slept much last night and wasn't thinking clearly. Funny though, I did sleep through the night.

I get so frustrated, agitated, and defensive when I mess up!

Sometimes I think I am losing my mind. Went to the mall today, my day off. Had a glorious morning shopping—a seldom treat. Took advantage of checking off all the necessities on my list. Too many bags to carry, tired and ready to go home when I can't remember where I parked my car. No clue whatsoever. Spent two hours wandering through the parking lot with no luck. Took the bus home. Came back with my husband at his suggestion when the mall closed to spot the car as the parking lot cleared.

This just isn't normal. Everyone forgets where the car is parked from time to time but I've never known anyone to need help finding it. She clearly is not right. My wife was always on top of everything. Could keep up with four schedules, the house and a demanding job and now she can't find our car? She promised she'd see the doctor. I think she is stressed....

Stage 3

Life goes on but it is now so hard to keep it all together. People during this stage generally continue to work, arrive on time, continue to be involved in favorite leisure activities; however, strategies that have always worked before begin to crumble. The effort to keep everything together is almost overwhelming.

I don't believe I have dementia, but would like to share an event that happened to me, which may explain what life at Stage 3 might resemble.

As a clinical consultant for a rehab company, my job requires me to be on the road most days and travel as many as 6,000 miles in a month. One of the benefits of my employment is use of a company car. Now, for many people a car holds major significance. I know people who love their cars. They will wash them; they even name them. I am not one of these people. For me, if you put the key in the ignition and it starts, it's a great car.

My family and close friends know that I am a bit quirky. I have an extreme fear of driving over water. My phobia has always been that my car would plunge over the bridge and into the water and that I would be unable to get out as the power windows and locks would not work. One of the contracts that our company was providing rehab services to at that time was located in Nassawadox, a small village located across a twenty-plus mile bridge. My company, knowing how I felt about going over large bodies of water, decided to provide a new car with manual windows and manual door locks.

As stated earlier, I am a bit quirky. I generally have only one route to any given location and will use this route every time unless something, like road construction, forces me to change. Although I am hardly ever there, my company has established office space in a building located in Lynchburg,

Virginia. For those of you who have never had the pleasure, Lynchburg is a beautiful city, but for me it follows no plan or reason on how the streets are laid out. I have one way of finding the Lynchburg office and have not attempted to find another. One morning while working at this office, my co-worker suggested that I check out a new store at the Lynchburg mall. I had never attempted to find the mall; however, it seemed that today should be my first attempt. I followed my friend's directions to the letter and soon found myself at the mall. I parked my car, went into the mall, and found the desired store. Leaving the store, I realized that I had not been paying attention to where I was going and I couldn't remember which door I had used to enter the mall. Once out of the mall, I had no idea where I had parked the car. Unfortunately, the story gets worse as I had the new car and I didn't remember what color it was or what the license plate number was and I had not written it on my hand.

As a clinical consultant requiring me to provide resources to almost 100 clinicians throughout Maryland, Virginia, and North Carolina, my car is always stuffed with boxes, papers, and assorted rehab equipment.

So I had only one strategy available to me that warm summer afternoon. I began to walk up and down row upon row of cars, looking for a new car with manual windows and filled to the top with resources. After about an hour, I found a car that fit these criteria. I placed the key in the lock and the door opened. What was only to be a quick trip to the mall had turned into a two-hour ordeal. I believe the way I felt for that short two-hour period is much like what people in Stage 3 feel all the time. Their compensatory strategies are no longer covering their memory losses and people are starting to notice.

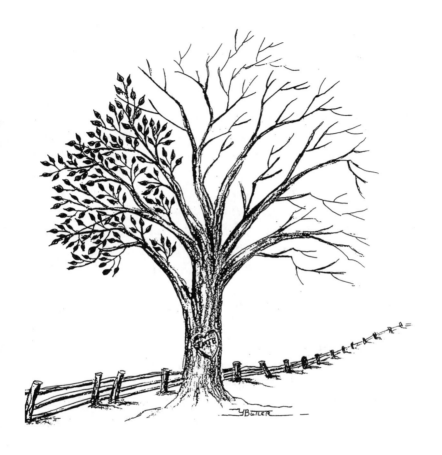

STAGE 4

People act strange around me. I can't find my way to the store. What am I going to do? I don't want to be a burden. I don't want to miss my daughter's wedding, my son's graduation. I want to enjoy my grandkids. I know I am not right. My life is over. This is no life....

A call from the doctor has just confirmed my worst fear. My wife has a dementing illness, possibly Alzheimer's disease. My God, she is only forty-five years old. We have been married twenty-three years. It has not always been easy—some give, some take, but I always thought we'd be one of those couples who had the tacky fiftieth wedding anniversary party with family, friends, cake, and pictures. My whole world has come tumbling down.

Alzheimer's Disease—What will this mean? How do we tell the kids? They've been asking lately, "Do you think Mom is all right? She seems so preoccupied, at times distant, at times frustrated and testy for no apparent reason."

I thought she was stressed—what with the demanding job and active teenagers. Strange though, things I wrote off as stress are racing through my head—the lost car, the repeated questions, the frustration.

Just checked the stove. I now have to be certain it has been turned off. She left the oil heating in a pan. Loves fresh popped popcorn but got sidetracked and never completed the job. She's no longer able to work and I'm not able to leave her side.

Stage 4

Residual memory is a powerful force. We go about our lives and never think how many of our everyday tasks and activities are completed sub-consciously, never realizing that we are doing them exactly the same way each time.

Where you place objects in your home is unique to you. Many of my favorite memories surround activities that occurred in the kitchen as I was growing up. Entering the kitchen you would pass a massive refrigerator and directly after this refrigerator was a cupboard which contained water glasses and coffee cups. When I left home to continue my education I did not think much about where objects were placed in my new apartment, I simply put them where they seemed to belong. As the years passed, I continued to move and rent several apartments and houses. Each move required me to relocate all my worldly possessions, but again, little thought went into where they should be placed, I simply placed them where they seemed to belong. It was quite amazing when I started to analyze where I had placed each object in every apartment and home that I had lived in. The coffee cups were always placed in the cup-board directly after the refrigerator.

Recently my parents sold their home and moved into an apartment. On my first visit to their new home, I walked past their new refrigerator, and reached into the first cupboard for a coffee cup and found one. My mother, seeing me do this, was amazed and asked how I knew the coffee cups were located there. I said they had always been located there, and then proceeded to point out where the silverware should be, where the oven mitts should be located, where the pots and pans should be located and, to her amazement, in every case I was right. We are creatures of habit, and we tend to fall back to our residual memories.

To demonstrate the power of residual memory, I will use a personal example. Almost ten years ago my wife and I built our dream house. The house has a very open floor plan and a very large kitchen, as the kitchen still holds a significant place in our lives. As we are both occupational therapists, part of what we do professionally is to look at energy conservation and work simplification techniques to make everyday activities as easy on the body as possible. As we developed the floor plan for our house and looked at the set-up of the kitchen, we decided to place the plates, cups, and glasses next to the sink and dishwasher to improve efficiency. Every morning for the past ten years, I have walked into the kitchen, passed the refrigerator, and looked for a coffee cup in the cupboard directly after it. We have never had coffee cups located there in this kitchen!

A number of years ago I assumed the position of supervisor of Occupational Therapy for the Adult Rehabilitation Unit at the University of Virginia. The adult rehab unit consisted of twenty-two rehab beds, and ten specialized beds for geriatric rehabilitation. Due to my love of the elderly, often I chose to treat patients admitted for rehab on this unit.

In order to be reimbursed as a free standing rehabilitation unit, insurance companies and Medicare required progress to occur in two disciplines (occupational therapy, physical therapy, or speech and language pathology) within a two-week period.

One of my job duties as supervisor of occupational therapy was to justify and hire new occupational therapy staff. I attempted to hire staff from occupational therapy programs throughout the United States. I believed by doing so we would obtain diversity in our approach to treatment, thereby providing our patients with the very best treatment possible. Even with this diversity of approach to treatment, all of the therapists were forced to discharge their confused, memory impaired geriatric clients to long-term care facilities, as they were not making measurable progress, and it was felt that it would not be safe to discharge them back to their prior living arrangement.

While working for the University of Virginia, I had the good fortune to do a clinical exchange with a large hospital in Glasgow, Scotland. The university's adult rehab unit was planning a new head trauma unit and as the Glasgow Coma Scale was developed at Southern General Hospital, I felt that the Scottish approach to head trauma might benefit us in developing our program.

I found health care in Scotland to be very different than in the United States. Prior to discharge from the hospital, all patients were assessed in their home environment by having a home visit. It didn't matter if the home or flat was located in Glasgow or three hours away in the highlands, a visit was scheduled. Many of my clients in Scotland displayed memory problems—unable to remember conversations that had occurred only minutes before. Although I felt that these individuals had little chance of returning home, I scheduled their home visits and accompanied them across Scotland to their homes. What occurred when we arrived at their homes truly amazed me. It was as if a blanket of confusion was removed from them. The individual who could not remember even the simplest new tasks would ask me if they could make me a pot of tea. They then would show me where all their worldly possessions were stored. As a result of this observation, the adult rehab unit at the University of Virginia instituted a new policy, which required therapists to complete home visit assessments with all confused clients within a fifty-mile radius of Charlottesville, Virginia.

Many families become aware for the first time that their loved one has a problem with their memory during Stage 4 on the GDS. Prior to this stage the individual does such a good job of hiding their confusion that family, friends, and co-workers are unaware of the extent of cognitive impairment. However, the individual realizes that compensatory strategies are no longer trustworthy and fears what will happen when he/she can no longer remember and safely live at home.

Throughout my professional career while working with people with memory impairment and their families, I have found that although each scenario is different, a common theme often occurs. The son or daughter will call mom/dad and say they are coming over for a visit. Mom will put on the coffee pot or teakettle in anticipation of the visit. She then decides to quickly vacuum the rug before the family arrives. When the son/daughter arrives, they discover the teakettle has burned dry while their mother continued to clean, unaware of the status of the teakettle. For the first time the realization that mom or dad may not be safe living alone becomes a reality.

Family members now have a major dilemma. Where do they place their family member? Many children attempt to move their parents into their home to provide a safe environment. All too often the confusion increases. It has been noted that during this stage people often have periods of becoming lost in space. Although they have lived in the same city or on the same street for fifty years, they become lost only blocks away from their home. It is as if they have been dropped into the middle of Tokyo, Japan, unable to locate common landmarks. Fear by family members that the individual will wander away from home and become lost increases throughout Stage 4 GDS.

Individuals in Stage 4 GDS dementia realize they are having problems with their memory. They realize they are asking the same questions time after time. They just can't remember the answer. After asking four times throughout the day where the bathroom is located, they wait too long and are incontinent for the first time in their lives. They were ashamed to ask the same question a fifth time.

An interesting statistic shows that urinary incontinence is the second leading reason for admitting someone into assisted living or long-term care. Families will do just about anything for their loved ones. However, when a parent demonstrates urinary incontinence and there is the constant need for clothing changes and increased need for laundering bed linens, often a decision is made to look outside the household to provide assistance. The memory-impaired individual may become increasingly upset with family members. He/she has been forced by the children to leave the home where everything was familiar and compensatory strategies worked most of the time, and move into their children's home, where nothing seemed to be where it should be and strategies were continually breaking down. Facing a move into long-term care is now a possibility.

Is your home safe for your loved one with dementia?

Over the years Kari and I have been asked to look at the home environment and provide basic ideas on how to address this common problem. This is our attempt to do so.

An elegantly groomed woman stands on a countertop searching for cookies in the "goodies cabinet," falls off the counter and fractures her hip.

A retired surgeon, believing that his wife is an intruder, slashes her with a knife.

An emaciated eighty-nine-year-old wanders from her home, and police find her two days later, dehydrated, lying on a park bench.

Unrelated incidents? No, all of these behaviors may occur with someone who has dementia. Because individuals in Stage 4-7 of the Global Deterioration Scale may become confused or may lack judgment and often engage in impulsive and dangerous behavior, the home environment becomes a potential danger zone.

The following is an easy to use Yes/No checklist for behaviors:

1. Is the individual with dementia well groomed?
   a. Cleanliness
   b. Nails clean
   c. Body odor
2. Is the individual with dementia well nourished?
3. Can he/she feed themselves?
4. Is the individual continent? (wet or soiled)
5. What is the individual's emotional state? We often ask the family or caregiver to keep an hourly diary for two days, reporting any behavior or emotional outbursts.
6. Does the individual have a history of wandering, particularly at sundown?
7. Does the individual have a history of endangering him/or herself?

The following is a comprehensive checklist that includes six sections of the home. Each section has five questions/areas to assess.

Kitchen

- Stove burners covered, locks on oven doors/refrigerator (if needed)?
- Sharp items, glassware, electrical cords, and appliances locked in cabinets?
- Child-proofed, locked cabinets (especially those containing cleaning supplies and chemicals)?
- Garbage out of sight and reach?
- Secured water faucets? (Turn off water when caregivers are not using sink.)

Bathroom

- Medications locked up and out of reach?
- Grab rails in shower and by toilet? Mat, bath bench in tub?
- Sharps (razors, tweezers etc.) locked up in cabinets?
- Small area rugs removed?
- Water temperature lowered, faucets removed or water turned off?

Bedroom

- All sharp corners covered?
- Small slippery carpets/rugs removed
- Bed height accessible (not too high)?
- Clutter and small breakables removed?
- Heaters covered?

Stairway

- Gates installed?
- Clutter removed?
- Adequate lighting/non-glare (at top and bottom of stairway landing)?
- Stair edges marked and identifiable (preferably yellow)?
- Non-skid surface on stairs?

Living Room

- Movable furniture removed?
- Sharp corners on furniture covered?
- Adequate lighting?
- Clutter, breakables, and electrical cords removed?
- Poisonous houseplants removed?

Yard
- Fences around yard installed?
- Double locks on doors, entrance, and exits?
- Poisonous plants and hedges removed?
- Lawn tools, chemicals etc. locked up?
- Dangerous areas secured: Pool, stairs, woods, unlocked cars etc.?

Finding the Right Placement

Perhaps the most gut-wrenching aspect of care for someone with a dementing illness is the issue of proper placement. While it is possible to successfully set up a home for safe management, it is also possible to find exceptional care outside the home. The latter, however, will take careful consideration and thorough investigation. We like to suggest several items of investigation when looking for placement outside the home.

- First, ask for references from responsible parties of past and present clients.
- Second, check the environment. Once a facility is identified, make an unannounced initial visit to see how the staff reacts. Are they calm and professional? Are they pleasant and accommodating? Do they offer an appointment for a return visit and tour? If still interested, make surprise visits morning, noon, and night. Inspect the facility for cleanliness and check for odors that linger. Check out the lighting to make sure there is adequate lighting throughout the facility and check for natural lighting from window sources.

Is there access to safe use of outdoors? Look at the restroom. Is it easy to identify? And most importantly, is there a homey feel? Trust your observations and instincts.

- Third, educate yourself about the staff. Is there an administrator present? Ask to meet the attending physician. Ask about staff retention and staff to client ratios. Ask about licensed medical professional availability, i.e. dieticians, nurses, physical and occupational therapists. Ask about staff training on dementia. Look at the overall demeanor of the staff—do they appear happy and alert? Are they well groomed? Are they interested in those they are serving? Do they engage their clients in meaningful activity?

- Fourth, explore the dietary services. Look at sample menus and food trays. Is the food properly hot, cold, or appetizing. Are there adequate means of hydration? Are the clients feeding themselves or at least participating in a feeding program?

- Fifth, investigate leisure opportunities. Meet with the activities or recreational department. Are the clients actively involved in activities that are meaningful to them? Are activities happening? Look for client participation in the activity. Sitting in a circle having the newspaper read to them is seldom meaningful or conducive to participation, so perhaps an activity like planting a garden would indicate a facility with more dementia appropriate activities.

- Sixth, choose a place where physical and emotional well-being is emphasized. Ask about roommate selection. Ask about the average length of stay. Can your loved one transition as necessary to greater levels of care within the same room or facility? Inquire about pharmacology policies. Are difficult clients handled by medications too often? Is there an open visitation policy?

- Seventh, look at your own well-being. What support is available for the caregiver or the family? Are there family nights, family support groups, or opportunities to serve on family council committees? How does the facility plan to inform you of changes or incidents involving your loved one?

Exploring the above categories in any order will help you to eliminate facilities that are not conducive to Dementia Possible Care©.

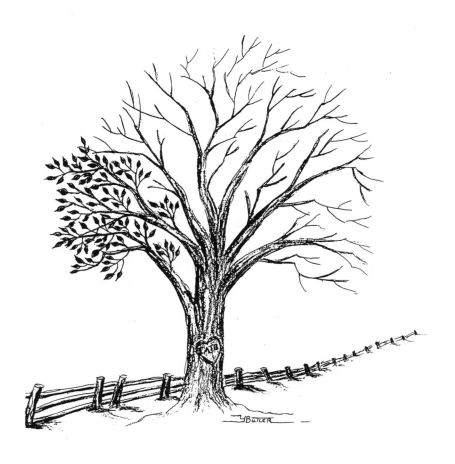

STAGE 5

I can't continue like this, she's losing her way in our neighborhood. Very social, beautiful, and well groomed as ever but she no longer even recognizes her own memory problem. I keep hiring caregivers so I can work but this has been extremely unreliable. Some call in sick, some don't understand the disease and mistreat my wife. I came home to find her soaked in urine today. Friends have stopped coming by, they just don't know what to say or do.

I believe I am beginning to accept that she can be better cared for outside of our home but I am guilt ridden.

I've visited several places. I was impressed with one because of the interaction I had with the staff. An occupational therapist shared with me that there are things that can be done to make her life meaningful. He suggested that we start by filling out a "My Way" form.

Stage 5

A "gift" of dementia is the fact that by Stage 5 on the Global Deterioration Scale the individual no longer realizes he/she has memory loss. People in this stage of dementia no longer agonize over what will happen when they no longer remember. They no longer worry about their past, nor do they fear the future, they once again LIVE.

An individual that demonstrates Stage 5 dementia looks just like you or me. They wear their clothing appropriately, they wear makeup, if they have glasses, they wear them. If they have dentures, they remain in the individual's mouth. In other words, on the surface, these people appear normal. However, the damage to the brain has progressed. These individuals have approximately five minutes of short-term memory.

Recently, I was visiting an assisted living special care facility in Maryland. I walked into the living room and was invited by a kind looking woman to sit for a minute on a sofa next to a roaring fire. She started our conversation by noting that I was new here and asked where I was from. I replied that I lived near Charlottesville, Virginia, and was just visiting today. She was thrilled; she stated that she had wonderful memories of Charlottesville and loved walking where Thomas Jefferson had trod. She said that the University of Virginia was one of her favorite sites to visit. I asked her where she lived and she stated that she lived in Washington, DC. She said she lived about two blocks from the National Cathedral. I asked her if she still drove a car. She replied that you would have to be a fool to drive in Washington, DC, given that they have an excellent Metro system. She talked at length about her favorite spots in the National Cathedral and approximately five minutes into this interesting conversation she was distracted by one of the residents of the assisted living facility. As she returned her gaze on me, her face lit up and she stated, "You are new here, where are you from?" This exact conversation continued almost word for word four more times in the next hour! I had no idea this woman had dementia; I assumed she was visiting a family member.

Caregivers who work with people who are confused, disoriented, and/or demonstrating short-term memory loss are special people. However, when faced with the same question twelve times an hour, often it starts to affect even the best caregiver. An example of this might be the person who asks every five minutes what time it is. I have seen even the best caregiver succumb to their frustration and say, "I told you twelve times what time it is! Stop asking me that question!" I often have to remind the caregiver that due to the resident's short-term memory loss they do not realize they have ever asked the question and can't understand why you seem so irritated with them for asking a very simple question.

A primary characteristic of Stage 5 individuals is that they never live in a long-term care facility; rather, they are just visiting. They will fabricate elaborate stories about how they volunteer in this facility to help "these poor individuals."

People in Stage 5 dementia are an activity director's dream come true. They want to participate in every activity planned. But not only do they want to participate; they want everyone else to benefit as well. Often you will see two individuals walking down the hallway hand in hand. This duo can be two females, two males, or any combination thereof. If you look very closely, you will note that one of the individuals is a step or two ahead of the other. The person in front is in Stage 5; the other usually is someone in Stage 6 dementia.

People in Stage 5 dementia should be 100 percent independent in all self-care activities. They may need signage to locate their belongings, but little else is necessary to maintain this independent status. Wording of signs is very important and very individual.

While consulting to a special care unit in an assisted living facility in Northern Virginia, I was asked to look at a new resident in the facility that was making great progress in her occupational therapy program. The therapist had labeled all dresser drawers and closets with the objects located within. As I was looking at the extensive labeling, I noted that on the closet door was written the word "briefs." Now being a male, I know that underwear can be briefs or boxers, however, this was a female's room, and generally underwear is not stored in the clothes closet. I opened the closet and could not understand the significance of the sign. In the closet were dresses, coats, blouses, and slacks. I asked the therapist why he had placed this sign on the closet door. He replied that this individual had stress incontinence and wore adult incontinent pads, which were stored on the floor of the closet. I located one of the pads and asked the woman what the object was. She stated "big bloomers." The sign was changed by the therapist that day.

Generally the sign on a bathroom door should be labeled "Toilet." Remember, Stage 5 individuals are just visiting the facility and do not live there. When they see the bathroom in their room they assume this is not their bathroom but a public restroom. About fifty years ago the signs on public restrooms read TOILET.

As mentioned earlier, people in Stage 5 of the Global Deterioration Scale for dementia look normal. Social graces remain. During conversations, if the individual previously looked you in the eyes when speaking, this behavior continues. Their posture is normal, and their gait looks normal with a natural step length and cadence.

Escape behavior will occur more frequently in the first thirty days in a long-term care facility than any other time with Stage 5 residents. It is essential that caregivers know all the residents of their facilities, as Stage 5 individuals look like they are visitors. As a consultant, I visit new facilities on almost a daily basis. Over the years I have been asked by hundreds of individuals if I knew where the door to the outside was. They would explain how they were visiting their friend, or husband/wife, and as all the doors looked the same they had become lost within the building. I often became confused while in the new facilities myself, so I would find the entrance and escort the individual to the door. Later I would discover that I had aided the escape of a new resident of the facility! Now when approached, I will escort the individual to the nurse on duty only to find that indeed, they are just visiting family members. Better safe than sorry!

What do we do if a resident elopes from the special care dementia unit/building?

The first method is to use the information that you know about the resident. Most residents who elope are trying to return home to family and friends. Once out of the facility, a caregiver should approach the escapee and gently try to take their hand and bring them back into the building. As this encounter is occurring, a second caregiver should approach the two and shout something like Hey! What are you doing! Is he trying to rob you! Get out of here or I will call the police! As the first caregiver leaves, the second becomes the rescuer. The rescuer and resident slowly walk away from the facility. Approximately five minutes after the encounter, the first caregiver returns and states that the resident's husband is on the phone and asks if she would like to take the call. As this is the individual that the eloper is trying to get to, often they will immediately return to speak with their family member. When the individual returns to the living environment, the door can be locked to decrease chances for a new escape. When the individual gets to the phone it is explained that the husband, or family member, could not hold any longer. However, they were on the way to visit and would be there soon.

I believe the second method is much more humanistic. As an individual is admitted into the special care unit or assisted living facility, a request should be made of the family member to do a very simple audio message. The content of the message should be specific to what generally occurs in the home environment. An example might be something like the following: "Hi honey, I am running a bit late. I will stop at the grocery store and pick up the items you requested. I will see you in a few minutes. I love you." Every time the resident starts to get upset and tries to elope, caregivers can get the tape made by the family and say, "Oh, there you are, your husband just called and we could not find you but he left a message." Then you play the message, which generally will calm the resident. Due to the five-minute short term memory of people in Stage 5 dementia, the tape can be repeated time and again and each time it will be like the first time heard by the resident.

I have been fortunate throughout my life to meet exceptional people. There are people who, through only very brief interaction, have changed the direction of my thinking and direction of my clinical practice. One such individual is Naomi Feil. Ms. Feil developed a new approach to dealing with disorientation. My training as an occupational therapist had prepared me to deal with confusion and disorientation by using reality orientation. (Bringing the individual into my reality). The process to accomplish this task involved discussing the month, year, day, season, and weather. Ms. Feil's belief that you needed to enter the disoriented reality of the individual was, to say the least, thinking a bit outside of the box.

A workshop on validation therapy was the first continuing education program I attended post graduation from the University of North Dakota Occupational Therapy program. It so much affected my thinking that from that day forward it became my approach to dealing with confused, disoriented elderly.

Validation Therapy

The following is my attempt to summarize important concepts of Naomi Feil's validation therapy approach to dementia management.
- Each human is different and valuable, no matter how disoriented. Each stage in life has different goals, and there is a reason behind all behaviors.
- Disoriented elderly must tie up living to prepare for dying. They must restore the past to make

closure and to justify their lives. The disoriented residents have outlived their ability to defend themselves against losses and stay oriented. They have simply lived too long to cope with "reality." They feel they no longer conform to our rules.

- Validation therapy uses empathy (walking in the shoes of the resident) to build trust. Trust brings safety. Safety brings strength. Strength renews feelings of worth. Worth reduces stress. Some disoriented residents no longer need fantasy, as they now feel strong and worthwhile in present time. (Our time and reality.) Adult controls return. Speech improves. They begin to interact!

- Others choose to remain in the past.

- Validation means each person is different. Staff does not judge. Staff does not tell disoriented residents what they should do nor do they expect all residents to act alike. Rather, staff respects the unique differences in residents as each person responds differently to old age.

- Staff tune into feelings; listen to the residents; observe nonverbal behavior, and attempt to put the feelings of the residents into words to give dignity and to validate them as a person.

- Validation means respecting disoriented elderly who have lived a lifetime. Validation means to acknowledge their wisdom.

- We cannot tell the disoriented to "Stop living in the past...Play time is over!" Now the resident's life task is to review and relive past times. This is how they can justify having lived.

- Staff gives dignity back to the disoriented resident by validating their reminiscence.
- Alone, without validation, they vegetate.

In long-term care facilities, every day is the same as the last, with the exception of the activities presented. The significance of the day of the week varies by culture and past experience. An example of this phenomenon is that Saturday is observed as a day of religious worship in Judaism and some Christian denominations. Sunday is observed as the day of worship for most Christians. If a sermon is preached on Thursday afternoon, many of the demented residents think it is Sunday.

Validation and Dementia

To validate is to confirm the experience of another person. We believe the number one reason working with an individual with dementia is frustrating is that often caregivers try to make the person with dementia confirm their own (the caregiver's) experience. In fact, success can only be acquired by our confirming the experience of the person with dementia.

An example of this would be trying to get Elsie to enjoy gardening when she never gardened nor had a desire to garden in her entire life. Choose the activity that inspires Elsie—perhaps it is going for a walk. This would be a physical example of validation.

Now suppose while you were on your walk Elsie started crying and said, "My dog just died this morning." You know that Elsie hasn't had a pet for at least ten years. Instead of correcting Elsie or changing the subject, it would be most appropriate to say, "I'm sorry to hear that. Please tell me about your dog." This is an example of verbal validation. It is much more effective because it will give Elsie comfort in feeling that you empathize with her sadness. This is where she is in her reality and no amount of convincing will put her where you think she should be at any given moment. Trust and cooperation will be established when you validate her feelings and let go of your perceptions of how things should be.

We treated a client on one occasion that served in the army. When we asked her to stand up, she would stare at us blankly. If we said "Attention!" in a firm command, she would stand up immediately. Not only did she stand up, but she demonstrated the beautiful upright posture that she had while she was in the army. She was still in the army in her mind and we were able to accomplish transfers and gait as well as work on postural correction in this manner.

Our Five Steps to Validation

1. Go on a fact-finding mission. Ask yourself and everyone else who knows the person with dementia the following:

Where did he/she work, what were their job duties, what were their hobbies, their interests, their likes and dislikes, their favorite music, movies, TV shows, the names of children, spouse, pets, did they live through a depression, serve in the military, etc.?

2. Observe the person in action. Do not try to alter any behavior at the moment unless it is dangerous.

Watch; watch for a long time. Watch from a distance. Watch from a close proximity. Watch without trying to interpret—just observe. Check the person at various times throughout the day or night. Check the person's nighttime habits. Check in the morning as the person arises from bed. Check before, during, and after meals. Check morning versus afternoon and differing days of the week.

3. Observe the person in different environments. Try to include any environment that may be utilized in a daily routine. Observe in the bedroom, dining area, bathroom, and living area. Then get creative and observe them outdoors, at a restaurant, the mall, a baseball field, etc.

4. Now place yourself in their shoes. Try to imagine what they may be thinking or doing and assign meaning to their activity. It may take trial and error to come up with the ultimate answer but dare to get in there and start the process. For example, ask yourself: If I were Mabel, why would I be taking socks from other people's rooms? Do I fear I am going to run out of socks? Maybe. But further exploration reveals that Mabel worked for fifty years as a hosiery inspector at a mill. Perhaps she is inspecting the hosiery! This actually happened in one of our facilities and the solution was to give Mabel a basket of socks and hosiery to keep in her room for inspection whenever she got the whim.

5. Enter their reality. Do not try to structure their day around the way you think it should look, create their day as they see it. Encourage activities that have meaning to them to gain functional outcomes. For example, have someone hang clothes on a line to encourage standing, hold a pet if they love pets, wear a tie on Sunday if they have done so for the last fifty years, etc.

Let's use the example of Mabel taking socks and put it to the five steps of validation.

1. Go on a fact-finding mission. Mabel worked for fifty years at a hosiery mill where she inspected socks prior to wholesale. She took her job seriously and won numerous awards for the least number of errors in the quickest manner. She prided herself in her attendance and often shared that she had only missed five days due to illness in a fifty-year period.

2. Observe the person in action. Mabel is observed as she methodically goes to the rooms of other residents in the assisted living facility and collects socks. She deposits the socks on her bed and begins to inspect each one thoroughly.

3. Observe the person in different environments. Mabel only collects socks between the hours of 7:00 a.m. and 3:00 p.m. when she is on her living area. If she is engaged in a recreational activity in another location that she finds meaningful, some sort of craft, she does not try to gather socks.

4. Now place yourself in their shoes. As Mabel, you imagine that unless you are engaged in a meaningful activity other than work between 7:00 a.m. and 3:00 p.m., it must be a workday. You have a quota to meet and a reputation to uphold with regards to accuracy and attendance and you must get to work!

5. Enter their reality. You create a day where Mabel participates in group and individual recreation activities that are often craft oriented because of her long-time hobby of crafting. In her spare time, you provide her with a large basket of socks to sort and inspect in her room or at a station set up for her in another area of the facility.

Holidays

Holidays hold special memories for all of us. For many it is the special food we prepare together. For others it is the special way the table and home is decorated. Each of us has our own family traditions. Many who celebrate Christmas, as an example, open their gifts on Christmas Eve, while others wait until Christmas morning.

Throughout the years we have been asked for advice as to what families should do during holiday seasons with their loved ones who are now well into dementia. Often family members feel guilty if they do not bring their loved ones home. Yet, when home, they become upset with all the additional stimulation and have catastrophic outbursts. For the individual who is now in late Stage 5 or entering Stage 6, holidays can occur on any day as they are now relying on their residual memory for most activities. Our advice is to continue to celebrate as you always have. However, rather than attempting to bring your loved one into this celebration, have a separate celebration with them in their environment. Perhaps they can still help in the preparations for the day by making a special dish, or preparing table decorations. Choose carefully what is in the best interest of everyone and give yourself permission to do it without guilt.

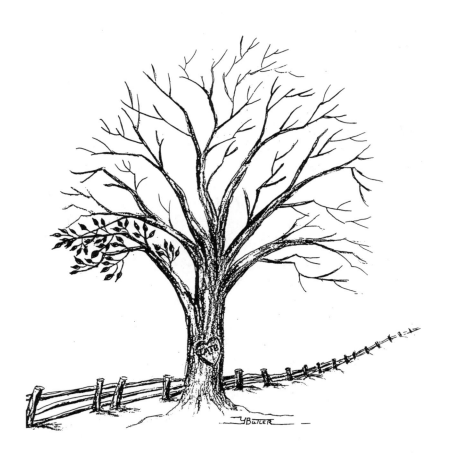

STAGE 6

Why won't she keep her shoes on? This is the third pair of glasses in two months. She's wearing diapers, how humiliating. My wife appears like a stranger—so disheveled. She wouldn't want to be seen like this.

The physical and occupational therapists have been instrumental in answering my questions and correcting the problems we have encountered. She kept her shoes on once we found a more properly fitting pair, seems she had a painful bunion that I was unaware of. I was surprised to find my wife was securing her glasses in a "safe place," her makeup bag, and the staff didn't have anything to do with the loss of her possessions. Gratefully, the OT discovered that she absolutely did not need diapers once a toileting schedule was established and the bathroom was labeled. The "My Way" form allowed my wife to continue to perform her own grooming and she began fixing her hair and applying her makeup just as she always had in the past.

I have put her in the right place. My time can be more meaningful with her now.

Stage 6

Perhaps my favorite client to work with is one who is in Stage 6 dementia on the Global Deterioration Scale. People in this category are like you and me at the end of a hard day; let's get comfortable. By appearance, generally, they look just a little off. Although still wearing all the trappings, subtle differences are noted. A man who has always worn a white shirt with a Windsor knotted tie, may still wear the tie, however, it no longer is centered and tied neatly within his collar. Glasses may only be worn for short periods of time and then discarded. Often glasses will be discarded because they are out of adjustment, or feel too tight to the individual's temples or ears. Dentures often disappear, never to be located again. This may be due to discomfort secondary to recent weight loss and change in fit due to atrophy of gum tissue. Nearly every long-term facility that I have visited has a box that contains a set of dentures with no idea as to whom they belong. Another common occurrence is to see a resident walking down a hallway with one shoe on and carrying the other. Almost everyone has one foot larger than the other. We tend not to buy our shoes in separate sizes to accommodate the differences, rather we make do and generally purchase them as a pair. If something does not feel right, or is uncomfortable, it usually gets removed by the resident during Stage 6.

Although little physical change may be noted by the untrained eye, a vast cognitive and marked physical metamorphosis is underway. Vision is beginning to change. As the person progresses into and through Stage 6 he/she will slowly lose their peripheral vision. Central vision will remain; however, side vision may become limited or non-existent. By the end of Stage 6, depth perception will be greatly affected. During Stage 6, people began to fall. A major reason for many of these falls is due to not knowing someone is approaching and when the person does come into their limited visual field they are startled and fall. Others, due to lack of depth perception, will over compensate their step height when crossing thresholds or change in flooring pattern and again lose their balance and fall. A third reason many people start to fall during Stage 6 is the fact that their stride length becomes shorter, they begin to shuffle their feet and catch their toes on the flooring. One of the common practices utilized by therapists is to put people who are prone to falls in rubber soled shoes. People with dementia and their shuffling walk will continue to catch their feet and stumble. It is extremely important not to place rubber soled shoes on dementia residents; leather soled shoes are a better choice.

A subtle difference between Stage 5 and Stage 6 is visual gaze. As mentioned previously, Stage 5 individuals look at the speaker during conversations. The eye gaze of the Stage 6 person will slowly progress downward until by the end of this stage it is about one to two feet in front of them. A functional impact as a result of this change in visual field location is that they tend not to visually track upwards, and therefore are unaware of most signage, as it is placed above their new visual field. It appears that approximately twenty to thirty inches from the floor is the ideal position for signs for this group.

I find that one of the favorite components of my job is assisting others in interpretation of behaviors. About a year ago, a new occupational therapist called me and informed that she was having great difficulty with one of her clients, as the resident was having frequent auditory hallucinations that were impacting the effectiveness of her treatment program. I said that I could be present during the treatment session scheduled at 8:00 a.m. the next morning and together we would attempt something that might improve her therapy outcome. The next morning, being an early riser, I arrived at the long-term care facility at 7:00 a.m. and proceeded to interview the caregivers on this resident's new behavior of auditory hallucinations. To my amazement, no one had noted that this resident was having this problem. I then arranged a meeting with the charge nurse and again was informed that the behavior had not been reported by anyone on staff. It was now almost eight o'clock so I walked into the dining room, our pre-arranged meeting spot. The client, whom we will call Minnie, was seated at a dining table, and the young therapist was standing off to one side of her. Upon my arrival the therapist issued the command for Minnie to eat. About ten seconds later Minnie said, "Momma, is that you, Momma?" The therapist looked at me and I shrugged my shoulders and the therapist repeated the command but this time with greater volume. "Minnie, eat!" Again after ten to fifteen seconds the resident stated, "Momma, is that you?" The therapist looked up at me and I stated that I did not think Minnie could see her. The therapist placed both hands on her hips and replied she had checked the resident's visual field and Minnie could see just fine. I nodded and again the therapist made the request but this time frustration was in her voice. "Minnie, eat your breakfast!" About ten seconds later Minnie stated with real love in her voice, "Oh, Momma, you want me to eat my breakfast." I said, "She does not see you, and I will prove it." Throughout the entire session, I had been standing quietly behind and slightly to the left of the table, well out of Minnie's visual field. I slowly walked up to the table and leaned down, moving slowly into the central visual field of Minnie. With a startle and a loud shout she exclaimed, "Did you just see that elf?" Being Norwegian, I do look like an elf or a troll, so again I requested that the therapist move into Minnie's visual field and make her request to eat. When the therapist complied, Minnie immediately began to feed herself. I later shared with the therapist the information that I had gathered from the caregiver staff earlier that morning. I believe Minnie's mother's voice must have been very similar to the therapist's. However, when the therapist moved into Minnie's visual field and made her request for her to eat, Minnie recognized that this was not her mother and simply followed the request. I often wonder how many demented residents are placed on psychotropic medication due to visual field deficits.

At one point in time, most individuals who are exhibiting the characteristics of Stage 6 dementia will stop feeding themselves. It is the responsibility of the caregivers to make sure that the residents eat and are properly hydrated. Therefore, when the resident stops feeding him/herself, the caregiver will began to feed the individual. It has been my experience that if you place a spoon in the resident's hand and provide two or three scooping movements with them, often the resident will continue the eating process. Many times we take away abilities from our residents without realizing they simply need a gentle nudge to continue.

While practicing as an occupational therapist at Southern General Hospital in Glasgow, Scotland, I was working with a memory-impaired woman in the central dining room. She had stopped feeding herself and I was trying to gently nudge her back into the scooping process by this hand over hand process described above. Southern General Hospital is run by nuns. Not the nuns as depicted in "The Sound of Music" or "The Flying Nun" on television, but STRICT Scottish nuns, who ran a tight ship and were proud of it. During the process of hand over hand with my patient, I heard two nuns talking. Their conversation went something like this: "Where is he from?" "Those are the worst manners I have ever seen." "One never fills one's spoon going towards oneself but always fills it going away." Realizing that I was the only HE in the room, I entered their conversation by stating that I was from the United States, North Dakota specifically, and we tended to follow our own rules of etiquette. However, as this individual was not making an attempt to begin feeding herself, I began to assist her in filling her spoon going away from herself. Within two scoops she began feeding herself! Now when I train new therapists and caregivers I remind them of this story and request if one method does not work, to try switching the direction of scooping, if that does not work, try to scoop on the diagonal, and if that does not work have them try with the other hand. About fifty years ago, when children started school, they were not allowed to use their left hand for activities in school. All activities, including eating, were completed with the right hand. As a result we have a lot of closet "lefties" out there. At some point they will begin to initiate self-feeding again during this stage.

Many occupational therapists, physical therapists, and caregivers fail to take the visual field of a demented resident into account when providing daily treatment techniques. An example of this is based on the initial training provided in our professional education programs. When an individual is using an assistive device, such as a walker or cane, often the therapist will position himself/herself to the involved side and slightly posterior to the involved leg. We provide added safety to the client by utilizing a gait belt, or holding to the back of the client's pants or garment. Throughout our therapy, we slowly wean away supervision and verbal cues; however, contact with the client generally remains until the treatment session is completed. For a client in Stage 6 dementia, this placement of the therapist makes him invisible to the client due to their lack of side vision; however, they know the therapist is present due to the constant cues they receive from the gait belt they are wearing. When the therapist is not present, often the resident will walk out of the assisted device (walker), as it has no meaning to them. Again, if someone has never learned to use a walker prior to becoming memory impaired it is new learning and therefore little carryover will occur unless the therapist utilizes creative strategies in their intervention to provide meaning to the assistive device.

In 1999, I was working in a long-term care facility with an eighty-three-year-old retired nurse. The nurse had moved into the facility about two years earlier, and now was functioning at Global Deterioration Scale Stage 6. She was very independent in her self-care, and ambulated without assistance throughout the nursing home. Unfortunately, she had a fall and severely fractured her right hip. She was admitted to the local university hospital and, due to the condition of the hip, required a total hip replacement. The results of the procedure were not as hoped for, and the surgeon requested that for the next 6-8 weeks she not bear weight on her right leg. This individual felt little to no pain as she had an exceedingly high threshold for pain. Due to her dementia, she also did not remember that she had fractured her hip nor that she was not to walk on the right leg. Therapists in the hospital saw her for one treatment session and discharged her. They noted her to be a very difficult, demented individual who was unable to follow their treatment requests. She returned to the nursing home and was referred to occupational and physical therapy. Therapy immediately began working with her, utilizing the following creative strategies. This resident once again was able to walk safely throughout the nursing facility.

We placed a 2 x 4-inch piece of hook Velcro directly onto the sole of the right foot and then placed her sock over it to hold it in place. We asked the client not to step "on the thistles," and since she remembered from her residual memory how uncomfortable it was to walk over thistles, we no longer had to prompt her not to step on her right foot. Next we modified a rolling walker by adding a walker basket. In the basket we placed a large number of medicine bottles filled with unsweetened candy. This woman had been a nurse for over forty years, and now she had a medicine cart. One thing we as therapists knew about nurses was that they generally do not leave their medications unattended. With this simple creative modification, we had a client who did not walk out of her walker; rather she went about the nursing home passing out medications for the next eight weeks, using this adapted walker and maintaining her toe-touch weight-bearing status.

Individuals in Global Deterioration Stage 6 dementia can continue to be extremely independent in completing self-care activities; however, they must do it "their way." At this point in the dementing process, new learning does not appear to occur even with constant repetition. This is one of the common fallacies of therapists and caregivers. They attempt to treat a person with dementia as they would with someone who sustained a traumatic head injury.

Stage 6 individuals will continue to be continent if you implement two very simple processes into their daily routine; scheduling toileting about one hour following every meal and using the ninety-second rule.

People in Stage 6 dementia generally do not hydrate themselves. Many times this is as a result of not being able to identify where the water or liquid is located. Often the majority of liquid is consumed during meals. What goes in must come out. Frequently the need to void occurs within an hour of meals.

Over thirty years ago, while working in a nursing home as an orderly, I discovered the ninety-second rule. It was one of my job requirements to bathe/shower and assist a number of residents to bed each evening. I would enter the resident's room, transfer the resident into a shower chair, gather towels, washcloths, pajamas, and grooming supplies. Then we were off to the shower room. About two feet into the hallway the resident would void or have a bowel movement! In our nursing home, housekeeping staff did not work the evening or night shifts. As I worked nights (due to attending the University of North Dakota's Occupational Therapy Program during the day), we took on the role of housekeeping staff. If accidents of incontinence occurred on our shift, we had to clean them up. Within the first week working the evening shift, I had a new name. I was known as "bucket boy." I would carry a bucket with me to place under the shower chair, and remarkably within ninety seconds the action would begin. I would empty the bucket and off we went to complete the bath/ shower. At this time in my professional life I did not analyze why this occurred, but now I realize that a shower chair is a toilet seat on wheels. The pressure against the resident's bottom is one of the earliest residual memories we all have. This memory started with toilet training! I have often wondered why people read in the bathroom. Many people are unable to initiate the process of voiding or having a bowel movement immediately, therefore, they will bring reading material with them. Again, generally it takes about ninety seconds to have this process start, but for many of us ninety seconds seems like forever. When reading, we generally are not focused on voiding or having a bowel movement, rather on the article or book we are reading and it just happens.

For caregivers and therapists, ninety seconds seems like an eternity to wait. Most caregivers give up at about forty-five seconds, transfer the resident off the toilet or bedside commode, and find that the resident has not initiated the activity. With no results, caregivers then rely on adult incontinence products as they feel nothing can be done.

Toilet hygiene is another area where we take away abilities from our residents. The amount of toilet paper you use, how you fold it, and how you use it is specific to you and you alone. Many times when you hand a large handful of toilet paper to an individual, they simply look at it and appear to do nothing. If you wait about ninety seconds you may see something very interesting. They will tear a small piece from the handful of tissue and use it! Actually there is a logical reason for this behavior. Over sixty years ago there was a paper shortage in the United States due to WWII.

After toileting a resident, caregivers are very good about washing their hands. Many times, however, to assist the resident they are toileting, they will wet a washcloth and hand it to the demented individual. Caregivers often seem surprised when the resident begins to wash his/her face rather than their hands. If you handed me a washcloth out of the blue I would probably throw it at you as I tend not to use them and it is not part of "My Way" of doing things. Many caregivers have been amazed at what happens when after toileting they have placed the individual in front of a sink with a bar of soap and a towel. The individual will spontaneously wash their hands without verbal direction.

Toileting Tips

Dementia can wreak havoc when it comes to toileting skills. We have had clients who had bowel movements in the waste paper basket, clients who attempted to hand their caregiver feces, clients that would urinate in their closet or sink, and clients that would drink out of the toilet.

Let's step back and assess why these behaviors become prevalent with this population. We believe for the most part that clients who void in the trashcan have not been able to distinguish where the toilet was located. This often occurs when someone has been moved to a new location such as a family member's home or a long-term care facility. Remember the example of the closet door located adjacent to the identical bathroom door? When they can't locate the toilet, they go to the next best place—the sink, closet, or the trashcan. As for the woman that attempted to hand us her feces, she had been constipated for some time and we believe she was trying to show us she had had some success. As for the clients drinking out of the toilets—they're just thirsty. They go where they can identify water.

With careful observation and anticipation of behaviors of the person suffering from dementia, these situations can be effectively avoided. For instance, how can you make the toilet easier to identify? Can you remove the door to the restroom? Can you place a sign stating TOILET on the door? People with dementia often retain their ability to read well into the late stages. Pick a word that is meaningful to them. Think about the period of time when they grew up.

How were restrooms labeled at this time? Are they used to a symbol for male versus female? Did they use an outhouse with a half moon on the door? Make the toilet easy to identify once they're in the bathroom. Make the toilet in sharp contrast to the floor. For example, use dark green flooring around a white toilet. As for the woman who was constipated, this could have been prevented through diet, hydration, exercise, and a toileting schedule. People with dementia need to be reminded to go to the restroom. Remind them or physically assist them to the restroom every two hours during waking hours. As for drinking out of the toilet, offer more visible appropriate alternatives such as clear glasses of water sitting on the bathroom counter and about the living area where they can be readily found.

Observation of the behavior and interpretation of the meaning of the behavior will allow you to anticipate and prevent the behavior or use the behavior to your advantage.

Also, remember the importance of good lighting and the environmental conditions. For example, no spills to slip on and the ease of the management of clothing. Keep in mind that other aging conditions like poor vision and loss of fine motor control can make it difficult for the person with dementia to manage snaps, buttons, and zippers. Make clothing easy to manage without making dramatic changes to the type of clothing the person is accustomed to wearing. A big mistake we see family members make is replacing their loved one's old clothes with nice new ones to go to the nursing home or assisted living facility. The new clothes are unfamiliar and cause a new set of difficulties. If Myrtle has worn a dress for the past seventy years, don't try to put her in slacks!

Muscles Don't Get Dementia

Some may ask, medical professionals included, why bother with exercise for those with dementia. Our answer to this is that muscles don't get dementia! The physiological benefit remains—less frequent falls by increased lower extremity strength and balance reactions; better skin integrity by increased mobility, which means prevention of pressure sores; increased cardiovascular output and improved lung function preventing secondary issues like blood clots and pneumonia; improvement in bowel and bladder function; and increased bone strength by slowing or preventing osteoporosis, to name a few.

The psychosocial benefit remains—less agitation and frustration related to lack of mobility, dignity in the remaining ability to perform in a functional manner such as using the bathroom, and socialization with participation in activities.

So we've outlined the physical, psychological and social benefits of increasing and maintaining strength, but how do we go about it? While people in the early stages of dementia can participate in individual and group exercise activities, those in the latter stages require a more functional approach. Someone who does not have the capacity to follow instructions for exercise may have the ability to perform a residual skill such as climbing the stairs, squatting to pick up items that were "dropped on the floor," or walking through sand or grass for example. Creative interventions surrounding the individual's residual memories for personal interests like golfing or gardening should be considered.

There are numerous recreational/leisure activities that can be performed with residual memory. The key is that these activities must already be engrained as routine for an individual. While new learning for these activities will not occur, old learning may still hold. As a physical therapist, I have been able to help my clients gain functional progress through residual memory activities. An excellent example of this is dancing. Familiar music will often elicit residual dance skills. I have witnessed clients with a past fondness for dancing dance beautifully even though walking shows a gait pattern disturbance or poor balance. One gentleman could not stand up and balance on his own but could spin me around the room every time he heard polka music. This became our avenue to work on his balance. Dance brings a means for physical fitness including balance, strength, and endurance as well as a social component to our clients. More importantly, dance gives a feeling of pure joy and is an excellent stress reliever. Try music from the era of those you are working with and don't forget that dancing can also occur from a chair or wheelchair.

The list of residual recreational/leisure activities can be infinite. The following is a list to generate ideas to use with your loved ones or those you serve: fishing, cooking, gardening, cleaning, reading, rocking a baby, riding a horse, golfing, looking at photos, dining out, sewing, knitting, crocheting, and reminiscing. As you can see, these activities have benefits far reaching to provide cognitive, fine motor, gross motor, balance, coordination, stress reduction, and socialization. Pick an activity that will give the benefit you wish to achieve. For example, to fish requires fine motor dexterity to bait the hook or remove a fish. Balance and coordination are required to cast the line. Upper extremity strength is utilized to hold the pole or reel in the line. The person with dementia enjoys the socialization and exhilaration experienced on this type of familiar outing.

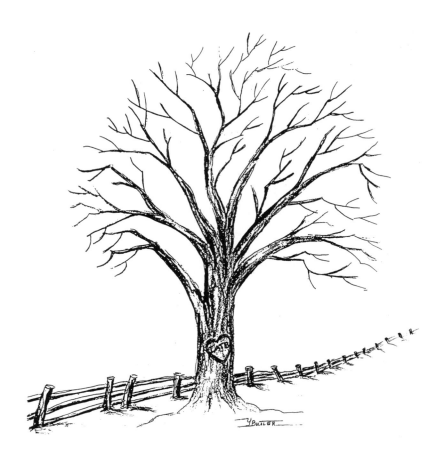

STAGE 7

It's been a wonderful journey. All she wants to do is snuggle. All those years she wanted to but no time. Life is complete again. We enjoy reminiscing about past times together. I remember things from long ago, like the way she would cross her feet as she still does now. Sometimes it seems she's not even here, then... she looks at me with the love and adoration I saw the first time we kissed.

Stage 7

We have entered the last stage of the Global Deterioration Scale and we now don't know what our loved one knows or what they no longer know. We do know that it has been an amazing journey filled with love, periods of great joy, and extreme sadness for us, as we mourn the person we once knew. We live for the brief moments of recognition, the instantaneous infectious smile of our loved one, the quiet moments spent together.

There is much we can anticipate during this period of dementia. How we deal with the process may dictate how your loved one progresses through this stage.

Many of our loved ones will stop speaking during this period of dementia. Some will revert to languages long deserted after being forced to use English at work and school. Others will mix English and their "native" language in their daily interactions with others.

Stage 7 appears to be a time where the senses once again dominate daily life. If something looks good, smells good, tastes good, feels good or sounds interesting, the individual will try to obtain it. We once talked with the husband of one of the residents on a dementia special care unit who shared with us that when he first met his wife they spent hours just sitting together and holding each other, not needing to speak. After they married, their jobs, children, and other demands they placed on themselves took the place of this quiet, wonderful time. Now, he stated, we can return to that treasured time together, no longer needing to speak, but just existing for the moment... together.

We spend much of our professional lives explaining to others that many behaviors people with a dementing disease exhibit can easily be explained. An example of this might be when our loved one no longer demonstrates an interest in food. We know that most people in end-stage dementia will die of aspiration pneumonia. Eventually our loved one will forget how to protect their airway and food will penetrate the air passages. Because we realize this to be a possibility, healthcare workers, doctors, therapists, and family members change the consistency of food to enable the individual to swallow it with a better chance of a safe swallow. As we change the consistency of food from whole to blenderized, the physical characteristics change. No longer does the individual with dementia recognize the food as food. Rather, they see a brown blob, a green blob, and a yellow blob of something on their plate. Often, we are unable to convince our loved one to even taste the new textured food.

Research has shown that as we naturally age, the last taste receptors we will have are the perception of something sweet and bitter. All other receptors slowly fade away. To ensure that your loved one continues to eat, we recommend that you never place blended food on a plate, but rather, place each food item into a separate bowl. When you serve the food, provide it one bowl at a time and call it thick soup. All blended food should be covered with sugar. Sugar over potatoes, sugar over vegetables, and sugar over the blended meat. If the individual has diabetes, put Nutrasweet or Splenda over the food, not Saccharin, as Saccharin has an aftertaste. Foods in their natural form may be best. An example of this is a banana. If given partially peeled and well ripened, you may find that your loved one has no problem initiating eating, and if they choose to walk away from the table, bananas tend to go with them.

When Kari and I travel as consultants to nursing homes and assisted living facilities, we often stop at other facilities in the area that we have never visited before. Generally we request to speak with the administrator or director of nursing and give them a yellow feather duster with our names and phone numbers attached. We suggest they call us and discuss the power of the feather duster and how we use it when providing Dementia Possible Care©. When they call we tell them the following story.

Some years ago, we were working in a nursing home with a special care unit for dementia. Each day as we worked on the special care unit, we could not help but notice a woman who visited her mother around 7:00 a.m. She would sit and talk with her mother for about an hour and then kiss her good-bye and leave for work. One day we noticed that the interaction between mother and daughter had changed. The mother had stopped talking over the past month and as a result the daughter now would arrive at 7:00 and, standing over her mother, start a conversation with her caregiver. The conversation went something like this: "How did Mom sleep last night? Did she have any falls? Has she had anything to eat today?" After this brief interaction with the caregiver, she leaned down and kissed her mother goodbye and left the special care unit. After observing this interaction, Kari and I requested doctor's orders for therapy as this woman now demonstrated a significant change in functional abilities and was no longer speaking. Our first interaction with this woman was to give her an apron with large pockets. We did so because I remembered how my grandmother had always worn an apron when in her home. It was almost a uniform for her as she put it on the first thing each morning and only removed it when she left the house to shop or go to church. One of the common behaviors of individuals with dementia is picking up objects within their environment and carrying their newfound treasures. By providing an apron with large pockets the client now had a place to save her treasures.

Earlier, we mentioned that when an individual enters the seventh stage of dementia they appear to be dominated by their senses. They appear to crave stimulation and if not provided to them they find their own outlets to fulfill this need. We gave this client a yellow feather duster. We chose the color yellow as that is the color we all see most clearly as we naturally age. This woman immediately began to rub her hand against the feather duster and marched down the hallway. At about 7:00 the next morning we heard the special care unit door open, then a low sob. The daughter had arrived and the first words out of her mouth were, "Mom, I didn't know you still could dust!" Mom had not changed; she still was in Stage 7 in her dementia, she still was not speaking. However, her daughter sat and talked with her mother for over an hour, reminiscing on what a wonderful mother and housekeeper she had always been. The power of the feather duster...the power of a new perception of her mother's abilities and a new reality of dementia.

Appendix 1

"My Way"
An Advance Directive

To Whom it may concern:
In the event that I should become cognitively impaired, I wish to record my preferences:

1. Sleep/Wake Cycle.
I maintain the following overall schedule:

Time I usually arise: _____

Nap times: _____

Time I usually go to bed: _____

Rely on clock to wake up   ___Yes   ___No

My side of the bed is   ___Right ___Left

2. Self-care routines.
I am accustomed to doing the following activities in the order indicated (1 = the first activity I do upon arising. 2 = the second etc.)

_____ Bathe   _____ Read the paper

_____ Brush my teeth   _____ Shave

_____ Comb my hair   _____ Use the toilet

_____ Apply make-up

_____ Dress

_____ Eat breakfast

_____ Make/drink a cup of coffee

_____ Feed the pets/animals

_____ Take medication(s)

_____ Watch TV news/weather/sports

3. Bathing.

My bathing preferences are (check those that apply):

a. ___ Shower   ___ Sponge Bath ___Tub Bath

b. ___ Morning   ___ Afternoon   ___ Evening

c. ___ Daily   ___ Every other day
     ___ Once/week ___ Less than once/week

d. ___Wash rag   ___ Sponge   Other (_____)

___ I never use same rag/sponge on face and groin/ feet
___ I never wash my face with the same water I sit in
___ I brush my teeth in the shower
___ I shave in the shower

e. I bathe my bodily parts in the order indicated (1 = first, 2 = second, etc.):
___ Arms
___ Feet
___ Groin
___ Back
___ Hair (head)
___ Chest
___ Face
___ Legs

4. Toileting.
Please check (and complete) your preferences:

___ I do not use public toilets
___ I use the toilet immediately upon arising in the morning
___ I get up ___times during the night to use the toilet
___ I don't believe in wasting toilet paper
___ I use lots of toilet paper
___ I fold the toilet paper neatly before use
___ I shut the bathroom door when I use the toilet
___ I need to sit awhile for my system to become active
___ When I "get the urge" I have to go "NOW"
___ I read while I sit on the toilet
___ I always stand when I urinate

5. Dressing/Undressing.
Please check (and circle) your preferences:

___ I sleep in the nude
___ I sleep in my underwear
___ I sleep in pajamas
___ I sleep in a nightshirt/nightgown
___ I stand while I dress
___ I sit while I dress
___ I put my (left/right) arm into cardigan-type garments first
___ When putting on cardigan-type garments, I put both hands in together & slip it over my head
___ I put my (left/right) foot into lower extremity garments first

___ I put on my (left/right) shoe first

___ Females: I hook my bra in the front of my body and then turn it to the back

___ Females: I hook my bra in the back

___ Females: I don't wear a bra

___ Females: I always wear nylons

___ Females: I always wear high-heeled shoes

___ Males: I wear (jockey style/boxer) underpants

6. Eating. Please check (and circle/complete) your preferences:

___ I never eat breakfast

___ I eat one food at a time and finish that food before I start another

___ I do not like my peas smashed into my mashed potatoes

___ I place my food in a particular arrangement on my plate (such as, meat at noon and vegetables at 3 o'clock)

___ I feed myself with my (left/right) hand

___ I prefer to sip liquids (before/during/after) my meal

___ I would gag if someone fed me

___ I cannot eat if someone near me chews with his/her mouth open

7. Occupation:

___ I worked outdoors
___ I worked indoors
___ Number of years in my occupation
Key elements of my job:

_____

_____

_____

8. Leisure/Hobbies

___ I enjoy inside activities
___ I enjoy outside activities
___ I would rather participate in group activities
___ I would rather participate in individual activities

9. Assistive Devices

___ Crutches
___ Cane
___ Walker
___ Braces
___ Splints
___ Corrective Shoes
___ Wheelchair

Appendix 2

THE GLOBAL DETERIORATION SCALE FOR ASSESSMENT OF PRIMARY DEGENERATIVE DEMENTIA

LEVEL	CLINICAL CHARACTERISTICS
1 No cognitive decline	No subjective complaints of memory deficit. No memory deficit evident on clinical interview.
2 Very mild cognitive decline (forgetfulness)	Subjective complaints of memory deficit, most frequently in following areas: (a) forgetting where one has placed familiar objects; (b) forgetting names one formerly knew well. No objective evidence of memory deficit on clinical interview. No objective deficits in employment or social situations. Appropriate concern with respect to symptomatology.
3 Mild cognitive decline (early confusional)	Earliest clear cut deficits. Manifestations in more than one of the following areas: (a) patient may have gotten lost when traveling to an unfamiliar location; (b) co-workers become aware of patient's relatively poor performance; (c) word and name finding deficit becomes evident to intimates; (d) patient may read a passage or a book and retain relatively little material; (e) patient may demonstrate decreased facility in remembering names upon introduction to new people; (f) patient may

	have lost or misplaced an object of value; (g) concentration deficit may be evident on clinical testing. Objective evidence of memory deficit obtained only with an intensive interview. Decreased performance in demanding employment and social settings. Denial begins to become manifest in patient. Mild to moderate anxiety accompanies symptoms.
4 Moderate cognitive decline (late confusional)	Clear cut deficit on careful clinical interview. Deficit manifest in following areas: (a) decreased knowledge of current and recent events; (b) may exhibit some deficit in memory of one's personal history; (c) concentration deficit elicited on serial subtractions; (d) decreased ability to travel, handle finances, etc. Frequently no deficit in following areas: (a) orientation to time and person; (b) recognition of familiar persons and faces; (c) ability to travel to familiar locations. Inability to perform complex tasks. Denial is dominant defense mechanism. Flattening of affect and withdrawal from challenging situations occur.
5 Moderately severe cognitive decline (early dementia)	Patient can no longer survive without some assistance. Patient is unable during interview to recall a major relevant aspect of their current lives. e.g. an address or telephone number of many years, the names of close family members (such as grandchildren), the name of the high school or college from which they gradu-

	ated. Frequently some disorientation to time (date, day of week, season, etc.) or to place. An educated person may have difficulty counting back from 40 by 4s or from 20 by 2s. Persons at this stage retain knowledge of many major facts regarding themselves and others. They invariably know their own names and generally know their spouses' and children's names. They require no assistance with toileting and eating, but may have some difficulty choosing the proper clothing to wear.
6 Severe cognitive decline (middle dementia)	May occasionally forget the name of the spouse upon whom they are entirely dependent for survival. Will be largely unaware of all recent events and experiences in their lives. Retain some knowledge of their past lives but this is very sketchy. Generally unaware of their surroundings, the year, the season, etc. May have difficulty counting from 10 both backward and sometimes forward. Will require some assistance with activities of daily living, e.g., may become incontinent, will require travel assistance but occasionally will display ability to familiar locations. Diurnal rhythm frequently disturbed. Almost always recall their own name. Frequently continue to be able to distinguish familiar from unfamiliar persons in their environment. Personality and emotional changes occur. These are quite variable and include: (a) delusional behavior, e.g., patients may

	accuse their spouse of being an impostor, may talk to imaginary figures in the environment, or to their own reflection in the mirror; (b) obsessive symptoms e.g., person may continually repeat simple cleaning activities; (c) anxiety symptoms, agitation, and even previously nonexistent violent behavior may occur; (d) cognitive abulla, i.e., loss of willpower because an individual cannot carry a thought long enough to determine a purposeful course of action.
7 Very Severe cognitive decline (late dementia)	All verbal abilities are lost. Frequently there is no speech at all – only grunting. Incontinent of urine, requires assistance toileting and feeding. Lose basic psychomotor skills, e.g., ability to walk. The brain appears to no longer be able to tell the body what to do. Generalized and cortical neurologic signs and symptoms are frequently present.

Global Deterioration Scale
B. Reisburg, S. H. Ferris, M. J. DeLeon, and T. Cook

About the Authors

Lanny D. Butler, MS, OTR, received his undergraduate degree in Occupational Therapy from the University of North Dakota and his advanced degree from the University of Puget Sound, in Tacoma, Washington. He has worked as an educator, consultant, and therapist for thirty years. The past sixteen years have been dedicated to serving the elderly. He researched and developed a practical approach to caring for individuals with dementia, called Dementia Possible Care©, and is the founder of IATB Dementia Care, a consulting firm on Dementia Possible Caregiving. Lanny and his wife Diane live in Crozet, Virginia. They have two adult children, Elisabeth and Andrew.

Kari Kent Brizendine, PT, graduated in 1984 from the Medical College of Virginia. She has had clinical, management, and teaching experience in a variety of settings including acute care, outpatient, and long term care, where she has cultivated her skills in the area of geriatric programming. Kari resides in Lynchburg, Virginia, with her husband Terry, daughter Katie, and son Kent.